BEING ICARUS

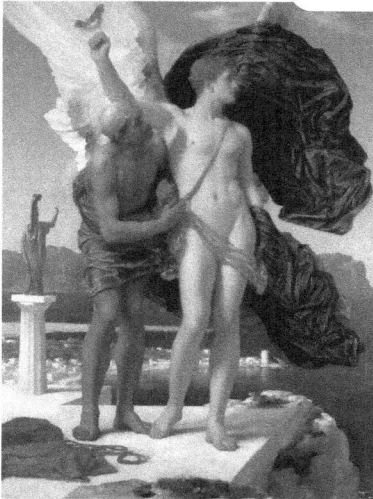

By Maureen Oliver

One million people commit suicide every year.
The World Health Organization

Maureen Oliver

Published by
Chipmunkapublishing
PO Box 6872
Brentwood
Essex CM13 1ZT
United Kingdom

http://www.chipmunkapublishing.com

Proof-read by Muna Hassan

Being Icarus

'...Icarus disobeyed his father's instructions and began soaring towards the Sun, rejoiced by the lift of his great sweeping wings. Presently, when Daedalus looked over his shoulder, he could no longer see Icarus; but scattered feathers floated on the waves below. The heat of the Sun had melted the wax, and Icarus had fallen into the Sea and drowned.'
From *Greek Myths*, by Robert Graves.

'In Breugal's Icarus, for instance, how everything turns away quite leisurely from the disaster; the ploughman may have heard the splash, the forsaken cry,But for him it was not an important failure; the sun shone as it had to on the white legs disappearing into the green Water; and the expensive delicate ship that must have seen something amazing, a boy falling out of the sky, had somewhere to get to and sailed calmly on.'
On Breughal's *The Fall of Icarus*, from *Musee de Beaux Arts*, by W H Auden.

Maureen Oliver

BEING ICARUS

Chapter 1.
With One Almighty Bound...

I clung desperately to the front of the massive intercity express. I was handcuffed to it by one hand and compared to the skyscraper-like proportions of the train I was the size of a flea. My friend Floris was handcuffed nearby. He shouted at me to brace myself should the train start to move. It was due to depart Amsterdam Central Station in about 60 seconds - bound for Vienna. I expected to die quite horribly, spattered like an insect against the speeding engine. For me, this was the latest in a series of near suicidal stunts that had become my trademark as a gay rights activist. I was 42 and, back in London I had left two teenage daughters to fend for themselves. What had led me, a previously shy, almost reclusive, artist to do this? It had all started two years before in 1987...

Autumn of 1987 - the great storm tore through the South London suburb where I lived with my children. I shivered in the darkness of that night as a mighty tree outside my window threatened to uproot and smash into the house. Clutching a birdcage with my children's budgies in it, I crouched on the carpet alongside the cat, and my dog, Bootie. It all seemed strangely symbolic, especially when I learned later that the eye of the storm had been a caravan park in East Sussex.

Maureen Oliver

My Mother's retreat, her much loved bolt hole, had been there and she had died in February; the destruction seemed meant.

It all seemed destruction that year, shattered by losing my mother I had to face the loss of my job in the summer. I had worked as a teacher running art and craft workshops in hospitals and day centres; I survived on part-time earnings and a tenuous contract. It was the '87 recession, and I fell victim to the cuts as my paid work simply ceased to be. I was a single mum, my children were bright and studying for college, I tried to get work but failed, things were looking very bleak. I was also a lesbian - a lonely one. Mum had been my best friend too. Needless to say, I cried a lot.

I started to take an interest in politics and human rights issues. An avowed feminist for many years, I became aware of the existence of groups campaigning for lesbian and gay equality. I visited a large and energetic meeting, and, seized with enthusiasm, joined an emerging group called the Organization for Lesbian and Gay Action - OLGA. Very shortly afterwards I found my way to a grimy office block in Farringdon, and, after a period as a 'tea girl', found myself in charge of running a campaign office. Now my life had purpose; I ceased weeping into my pillow every night and threw myself headlong into the gay political scene. I started by offering my skills as an artist, illustrating pamphlets and the like. Then Clause 28 happened.

I was walking back and forth outside the Houses of Parliament anxiously. I had been sent to talk to people demonstrating outside the imposing edifice. News of 'The Clause', a proposed government by-law that banned the 'promotion' of homosexuality by local authorities and, oddly, referred to the families of lesbian and gay people as 'pretended', had broken while I was busily photocopying flyers in the OLGA office. I had been asked to get down to the seat of government with alacrity to report on events. It was a chill, wet day and darkness had fallen early. All I could see were the usual desultory groups of tourists parading about. I could see no sign of any demonstration, all seemed to be business as usual. My anxiety levels reached fever pitch. If I returned to the office I would have to report failure. I panicked and decided to head for home. I started to cross Westminster Bridge, bound for Waterloo Station on the South Bank of the Thames. I was feeling unreasonably desperate. Then, a sudden compelling urge to leap off the bridge into the fetid waters below seized me. I was terrified, but I had to cross the river in order to get back to the sanctity of my suburban home. Absurdly, and to the amusement of passers by, I fell to my knees and crawled across the bridge. It felt safer that way. And so ended my first foray into activism -

ignominiously.

In the past, I had been dogged by depression. A depression that was relieved by periods of elation when I would paint through the night energetically while my children slept nearby, but so often I felt the keen edge of despair and would sob, write dreary poetry about death, and endlessly read the work of suicidal poet 'Sylvia Plath'. After a messy and painful relationship breakdown, I descended into a dark and lonely place. Finally, hallucinating and fearing I would harm the children, I attempted suicide and spent 6 months on a psychiatric ward. After my discharge I managed to regain custody of my kids and led a fairly quiet existence. This existence was not without problems however, I was still subject to mood swings and occasionally heard disembodied voices cursing and criticizing me. This was the self that crawled over Westminster Bridge that night and returned home in tears. It could have ended there, but it didn't - I bounced back.

I started by giving talks to small groups of people. Then, as my confidence increased, I mounted soapboxes up and down the country making speeches, fired with enthusiasm. I was interviewed by the press and began to be known as a vigorous and vocal activist. Somehow I had found the energy to throw myself back into the fray after that first distressing experience. My mood

BEING ICARUS

lifted. I became a political animal, leading marches proudly displaying my OLGA t-shirt. I took on more and more work. Back home, my two daughters, struggling with 'A' level exams and the vicissitudes of youth, had to cope without me.

When I joined OLGA, it was run by two liberated lesbians – Jenny and Lisa - women who were as camp in their dress and mannerisms as any overtly gay man, I call them liberated lesbians since they were definitely not of the same ilk as the lesbian feminists of my acquaintance. They wore make-up and dressed dramatically – Lisa had bobbed black hair and Jenny bleached blonde curls and their talk was of things unknown to me – sadomasochism, 'tops' and 'bottoms', bisexuality and 'cottaging'. I had come from the strictly politically correct background of the radical women's movement, and had absorbed the moral codes, and dress sense, of the feminists who played such a large part in the Greenham Common anti-nuclear protest. I wore dungarees, or loose fitting jeans, with men's shirts, and sported close-cropped hair. I hardly ever wore make-up – though occasionally dared a little mascara. My clothes, however, were not the uniform greys and blues, I was, after all, an artist and wore strong bright colours. A pair of yellow trousers I wore to the office one day prompted one particularly catty gay man to observe that I 'looked like a bowl of badly set custard'. I didn't wear them again. I was a sensitive soul. Jenny and Lisa came from a different world in other ways too. I had children and was a single mum – a lesbian mother – had no money and originated from a tough South-East London neighborhood, while they had unrepentantly middle class attitudes, an avowed interest in theatre, and regularly visited expensive restaurants and bars. On the positive side, they were imaginative and clever women. They used their abilities and their contacts in the theatrical world to good purpose. Early in the campaign OLGA organized an entire train to take hundreds of protestors to a massive rally in Manchester. The event proved a media triumph and the whole of Manchester was flooded with gay rights supporters. That night the clubs and bars were filled with happy homosexuals. Jenny and Lisa were, however, very 'single focused' in their views. For example, they didn't relate to the situation of lesbians struggling to bring up children in a hostile world. I had had first hand experience of that of course. The only thing we had in common was our sexuality, perhaps, after all, that should have been enough.

I remember the day the two of them decided to 'employ' me to run the office. In reality I was an unpaid volunteer. They promised to buy me a meal. I was excited at the prospect of being taken out to a restaurant by these worldly-wise women. We arrived at a small Italian café in Islington, the kind with red checked tablecloths and guttering candles alongside the ketchup and brown sauce. They asked me what I wanted and ordered it. To my horror I realized they were literally '*buying me a meal*'. They sat and watched me eat, smiling benignly, eating nothing themselves. This patronizing approach hurt me and I saw that to them I was a mere minion and of little account. Seeds of rebellion were sown in my heart that day. Jenny and Lisa would eventually be eliminated. I would become self appointed National Coordinator of OLGA, but, in the soft light of the café, as they talked of things strange and new, that was a long way off in the future and I kept my anger to myself.

Clause (later Section) 28 of the Local Government Act sent shock waves through the lesbian and gay community. Already demoralized and reeling from the impact of AIDS, and the insistence of the tabloid press on designating the disease a 'gay plague', we reacted with horror to legislation aimed at further silencing and alienating us from society. The intention of the Clause was to prevent the advertising and sponsoring of plays, books and exhibitions plus meetings and support groups. A howl of protest reverberated through a 'community' that had, until then, been a loosely knit collection of individuals and a few disparate groups. The great and the good offered their support to our campaign, for example, it was the Clause that precipitated the overdue 'coming out' of a venerable, nationally cherished actor – 'Sir John Gielgud' - and he was not alone. Actors, musicians and artists rallied to the cause, but for me, and for others like myself, it was that expression, 'pretended family relationships' that fuelled my fervour and made a frontline protester of me.

At first, I treated running the office as very much a job of work, getting up early and seeing the girls off to school before boarding a train for Farringdon in the City. I would go to a sandwich bar and buy a veggie sandwich at roughly the same time each day, open up the office and listen to the phone messages while I made a cup of coffee. That was how it started, but soon I was working like a demon, sleeping under my desk when I could, hardly having time even to change my clothes and in a frenzy of constant manic activity. Like the mythical Icarus I would try to fly to the Heavens but like him my wings were made of wax and would melt in the intense heat of the Sun – inevitably I'd plummet into the dark seas of despair. I was unaware of that fate however as I rushed around excitedly, motivated and fired with enthusiasm and revolutionary zeal.

My companion in the office was a disarmingly gentle and politically aware disabled gay man called Dennis Killin. We quickly became friends and I would often sleep in his Finsbury Park flat at

BEING ICARUS

night when I couldn't get home to far-flung Croydon. I developed a habit of stealing his clean underpants when I ran out of knickers, this caused him considerable annoyance, not to mention inconvenience, but Dennis and I quickly hit it off. Dennis had a visual impairment and other physical disabilities; the sight of Dennis and I, arms linked, at demonstrations and meetings was soon commonplace. We became firm friends as well as colleagues. I felt able to confide in him and told him about my previous psychiatric problems. In turn he introduced me to disability rights issues, and the wider world of political activism.

I attended disability rights events, anti racism meetings, the 24-hour picket of the South African Embassy (apartheid was still rampant then) and feminist rallies, I became known as a vociferous supporter of diverse causes, speaking on many platforms with conviction. I spread my net wide, taking on more and more commitments. Sleep began to seem like an indulgence, an unnecessary luxury and I saw myself as a vital link, building solidarity and rallying support. I put every ounce of my strength into my work. This would eventually prove a near fatal mistake.

Chapter 2.
Male/Female/Other

Then there were the women. I had always been a solitary figure. Having two teenage children was something of a passion killer for prospective lovers. My first fully intimate same-sex relationship had been wonderful but hideously cut short by my fear of losing my children. I had obtained custody via several bloody court appearances. That had been before my breakdown and subsequent incarceration in a mental hospital. In the eighties, many lesbians lost their children in vicious custody battles. Seen by the courts as 'unfit' mothers due to their errant sexuality, their kids were snatched away. Sometimes those kids ended up in the care of the local authority rather than with unorthodox, but loving parents. My partner, Jill, had been undergoing this process at the time. Although I empathized with her, my own situation, should I also be dragged into court, would be desperate. I was not only a lesbian but had a psychiatric history. Terrified of losing my daughters I abruptly severed my relationship with my lover. Afterwards, apart from the odd 'one night stand' there had been no more romantic or sexual encounters. All of this would change. Apparently being an effective speaker and campaigner was a powerful aphrodisiac. Women began to throw themselves at me with reckless abandon.

BEING ICARUS

There were women who offered to volunteer to work in the office then set about seducing me. I was up for seduction. As my mood heightened so did my sexual appetite. Many of these women were considerably younger than me, and this worried me a little, but who was I to turn down their advances? One particular woman was obsessed with the idea of having sex in the office and played the game of being my 'secretary' - that was OK by me, after all, I was having a whale of a time. Or was I? In a way there was something peculiarly impersonal about these relationships. These women didn't really know me; I was merely a figurehead. It was the vigorous campaigner they wanted, not the dreamer, the artist. They would approach me after I had spoken at a rally or meeting and invite me to their homes for a 'coffee'. I don't remember much coffee being drunk. Once I shared the bed of a woman who described herself as 'the voluptuous one' with her large shaggy black dog sprawled across it throughout the proceedings. There was a great deal of passion, but little love. I still felt lonely and isolated. And what had happened to the shy dreamer, the ethically conscious feminist - the loving mother? I was undergoing a metamorphosis of some kind.

And then there were the men. Gay men, my life became full of them, their lives, their hopes and dreams, their worries, their pain and the whole damned gay scene. Until about '87 I had been something of a feminist separatist and avoided all men. Then, one day in the local supermarket, I saw an exotic young creature, a man, or boy, dressed in red tights and a knee-length kilt – and full make-up. I thought to myself, 'he must be gay'. I was right of course, and soon, Stevie and I became firm friends. Stevie was an aspiring artist, I gave him support and encouragement and soon he became one of the family – a permanent fixture on the sofa in my living room. After I became involved with OLGA my world became choc-full of gay men. I grew to respect and trust them. Sometimes I trusted them a little too much forgetting perhaps that men are men after all.

In the summer of 1988 I travelled to Berlin to speak at a Women's Conference. The conference itself was fairly unremarkable, but afterwards one of the women took me to the Berlin Wall. This was, of course, before the Wall dividing East and West Berlin was torn down. The situation was still very tense; people were routinely killed trying to cross to the West. It was very dark and my friend gestured to me to climb a ladder propped against the Wall to take a look at East Berlin, and the border guards. She warned me though, not to put my head far above the parapet, as I could be shot dead. Nervously I peered over the Wall. East Berlin was uncannily silent and in complete and utter darkness, I was aware of the guards, their rifles at the ready. Behind me, West Berlin was a blaze of neon lights and colour and the streets were thronged with late night revellers. The contrast couldn't have been more extreme. I clambered down the ladder pretty quickly. It was a chilling experience and one I'll never forget.

I didn't fly home from Berlin but went instead to Delft in Holland. It was the day of Dutch Gay Pride and I was booked as a guest speaker. I was given a standing ovation by the assembled crowd of 7,000 and, tired but happy, set off to the house of a gay man named Dick who had promised to put me up for the night. I arrived at the house with my bag, feeling exhausted and longing for a bath and a bed. I knew Dick slightly; I had stayed at his house once before when I had spoken at the local Gay Centre on the evils of Clause 28 - and the worrying possibility of the Poll Tax. On that first occasion my visit to Dick's house had been pretty unremarkable, so I wasn't anticipating any problems when I knocked on the door of his charming little house in the heart of Delft. The door was opened by a man who was a total stranger to me and behind him were about half a dozen others. They were watching football on TV. The day of Dutch Gay Pride had clashed with a major football victory for Holland; the streets were full of joyful, drunken supporters, many of them with their faces loyally painted bright orange. The gay men in Dick's living room were obviously less interested in Pride than they were in football.

Maureen Oliver

Nervously I walked in, carrying my bag, and announced that I was a friend of Dick and had been invited to spend the night at his house. At that, one of the men grabbed me roughly and manhandled me outside while they all screamed threats and curses. Whether they thought I was a criminal or were just annoyed that I had interrupted the replay of the big match I didn't know, but I was out on the street, had no idea where Dick was, had no money and nowhere to stay the night.

A desperate few hours ensued. I went to a lesbian club where a party was going on. Here I eventually slumped to the floor - totally exhausted. Bizarrely, some of the women who had seen me speak at Pride were asking for my autograph while I crouched in a corner drained and weeping silently with sheer frustration. There was a language barrier. Though most Dutch people speak excellent English, everyone had been celebrating for hours and most were high as kites. However, a capable looking lesbian appeared at last, and she took me to some stewards at the door. She demanded that they find Dick and help me gain access to his house. After some considerable time, I was handed a set of keys to Dick's house, he hadn't bothered to come to my rescue himself. He was having too much of a good time touring the clubs and bars. When I finally got into the house, I found the football fans gone but

BEING ICARUS

the spare room occupied by a snoring man, I didn't feel happy about sleeping in Dick's big double bed, reasoning that he would be needing it pretty soon – and might not be returning alone. I tried to scrunch myself up into a small enough ball to sleep on his two-seater leather sofa, but it was impossible to sleep. I made myself hot drinks as the night wore on and began to have very negative thoughts about Dutch gay men – and men in general.

As dawn was coming up, Dick's key turned in the lock. He seemed surprised to see me on the sofa and said brusquely that I'd have to share his bed. He was alone but I naturally felt nervous about climbing into bed with him and so waited till he was asleep before lying down on the edge of the bed fully clothed. I awoke after a couple of hours, Dick was sleeping deeply, and I went downstairs to the kitchen area in search of some breakfast. Dick's other guest was there, tucking into slices of Gouda and bread and drinking coffee. He looked startled enough to faint at the sight of a woman emerging from Dick's bedroom, but I ignored his distress and helped myself to something to eat and drink. The guy hurried out and I took grim pleasure in imagining him contacting his friends with the news that Dick had spent the night with a female. About an hour later Dick surfaced looking almost as surprised as his friend. "Where did you sleep?" he asked. Obviously the festivities of the night before had obliterated his memory. "With you", I replied casually. "And nothing happened?" he said incredulously, "No-one sleeps in my bed and nothing happens!" I returned home soon afterwards, Dick drove me to the station and saw me off on the train. Ever afterwards I would refer to him as 'Dirty Dick from Delft'. A Dutch lesbian later commented, "That Dick, if a cat walked over his bed it wouldn't be safe."

Strangely enough, I encountered one or two gay men who seemed to have more than friendship in mind. Why did I warrant such perverse desire? After all, I was no Diva, just an ordinary woman and mother of teenage children who lived in an unfashionable London suburb. The secret aphrodisiac, I later realized, was that gift for public speaking – somehow my ability to hold and rally an audience made me desirable. Of course, all the attention went to my head. My spirit rose, like Icarus I unfurled my wings and started my flight. I found myself to be not only an effective campaigner but also curiously attractive – even to some gay men.

Of course most of my male friends were totally impervious to any sexual charms I might have and many of them became very good friends. Among those friends was Floris, reputedly a Dutch aristocrat, who lived in a beautiful seventeenth century house by the side of a canal in

BEING ICARUS

Amsterdam. I had met him on that first speaking engagement in Delft and we became very close. I spent some wonderful hours with him at his home, I could relax there and relaxation was a precious, and rare, commodity for me. Floris died in 1991 from AIDS and I still miss him.

Before I go any further I should explain something about my inner life. I was always someone who had a 'God shaped hole' inside. After spending my childhood and teenage years looking for faith, I became a Catholic at nineteen. It was a profound, life-changing experience. I would start every day by going to Mass at 7am. When I left Art College I worked in the bookshop attached to Westminster Cathedral – the catholic cathedral in Victoria. However, my unhappy and ill-fated marriage - we had wed at eighteen after knowing each other for only a few weeks - fell apart. After a beating I lost a baby. The relationship lasted another year but, at the age of twenty, I ran away with another man. Thus I fell foul of my church and found myself virtually excommunicated. I wept many bitter tears. In time, they would become tears of anger and resentment.

However, after my breakdown in 1980 I became a lesbian feminist and discovered the 'Ancient Religion of the Great Cosmic Mother of All', or so a book I was given described the Goddess. The idea of a female deity captured my imagination. I attended some meetings of a group called the 'Matriarchy Network' and embraced Paganism with enthusiasm. Goddess worship was associated with Witchcraft and soon I was studying books on the Occult. I began to read the Tarot, developed a passion for Astrology, Palmistry, Numerology, Candle Magic and all things arcane. I couldn't find a coven, but if I had done so, I would have joined up enthusiastically. All of this went some way to filling up the emptiness left by my Catholic faith, although I never totally relinquished it. Sometimes I would creep into the back of dark churches, say a Hail Mary and light a candle or two.

During my campaigning years, a few of the gay men I worked with began to call me a witch; I often did Tarot readings for them with uncanny accuracy.

My work running the OLGA office put me on the front line of the campaign. That summer, a national conference was planned. It was to take place in Edinburgh and delegates from all over the UK would be there to make vital decisions on policy. At the time, Jenny and Lisa were still titular heads of the organization – though they rarely came into the office. They saw the workers as unpaid 'staff' and kept their distance. They set the date of conference and we soon realized that this was the very day that a national rail strike was planned – we suspected a conspiracy. We believed they wanted to stop us from being at the conference at all. All three of us were extremely short on money and didn't have our own transport. The journey to Scotland would have been difficult enough for us, but with a rail strike planned it was beginning to seem impossible. However, we decided to take the overnight 'Stagecoach' bus – it would mean arriving at the conference sleepless and exhausted – but it was cheap and would get us there. A huge gulf had developed between the 'management' – Jenny and Lisa, and the 'workers' – Dennis, Ian and myself. We resented what we saw as their bourgeois attitudes and high-handed treatment of us. We felt we were not given the respect we deserved for all the hard work we did – and there was something of a political divide as well. Jenny and Lisa were 'liberals' and the workers held socialist convictions. We determined to have a powerful influence on that conference. Other 'dissidents' wanted to have their say too – a representative of the Black and Ethnic Minority 'Caucus' refused to attend a conference she saw as innately racist, and handed me a letter of censure to be read out in her absence.

On my arrival at the venue, I quickly took up position as the official chair – I expected this to be disputed – I hadn't been voted in – but there was not a murmur from the assembled delegates. The Black and Ethnic Minorities group had, in fact, boycotted the meeting – so I spoke to a sea of aggrieved white faces. When the discussion turned to what had been, and what could be achieved, the atmosphere warmed. I seemed to have some popularity with the members and when Jenny and Lisa, by this time rather disgruntled, attempted to usurp my position and have me stand down and be restricted to a minor role in the administration, I managed to turn the tables on them and they lost control of the organization. As they left the conference grim faced, I waved at them and said a cynical goodbye. The workers had triumphed. Soon afterward I would designate myself 'National Coordinator' thereby acquiring an official position as spokesperson for the campaign. I was in total control – or so I thought at the time...

BEING ICARUS

Chapter 3
The Bus Tour.

The wings of Icarus unfurled and lifted him skyward.

In the autumn of 1988 a group of Amsterdam hippies came up with the idea of a European bus tour in support of our struggle against the Clause. The bus would carry lesbian and gay activists, musicians and comedians, and would travel from city to city, raising awareness. I was asked to be the voice of the campaign and to take my place on stages and platforms in five countries and nine cities to rally support. I accepted eagerly. I left my children and travelled to Amsterdam with the loyal Dennis, to undertake the long drive to Switzerland and join the bus. The bus tour had started in Paris, and had not yet had a very good reception. Six of us were crammed into a car designed to hold four people – Dennis was squashed into a small space intended for hand luggage along with the inevitable ubiquitous, hippie accoutrement – a guitar. We drove through Belgium and part of Germany in intense discomfort and finally arrived at the Swiss Border. Here we were stopped by Border Guards at gunpoint and ordered out of the car - they searched it, presumably for drugs. A group of dishevelled, disreputable looking individuals on route from Amsterdam must have aroused intense suspicion. We endured a terrifying couple of hours. We were forced to stand stock still, our hands in the air, guns pointed at our heads. After the car had been ransacked, and we had been interrogated and searched, we were freed and allowed to cross the border. We travelled on to Basle – our belongings in a confused heap in the boot along with the, now broken, guitar. However, Basle was to prove something of a personal triumph...

By this time I had already notched up radio interviews and TV appearances, but there was nothing to beat the experience of being appreciated and applauded by a large crowd. In Basle the 'Stop the Clause' benefit was a massive affair. At least a thousand people were packed into the venue to dance to the lesbian band 'Mouth Almighty', laugh at the antics of a group of gay Manchester comedians and listen to me speak. I received a resounding ovation; now I had begun to fly high, and it felt good – so very, very good...

From Basle we traveled to Zurich, the bus was no tourist express but a battered old crate, without sanitation of any description, in danger of completely falling apart at any moment. It sported a large pink triangle on the side – a well recognized gay symbol which sometimes led to the vehicle being pelted with stones, eggs and anything else local homophobes could find to hand – and graffiti inviting us all to die of AIDS was sprayed over it. We had to stop for quite a while to get the filth cleaned off. The roadside was our toilet, finding any kind of washroom on the way was an incredible luxury and we quickly accustomed ourselves to a nomadic life.

By the time we reached Zurich we were becoming very heavy drinkers, while food was whatever we could scavenge along the way – usually bread and cheese. We found the city a strange place. It literally dripped with gold, and yet in the park were drug users begging for change, with haunted eyes and ragged clothes. Everything was so expensive - we were hard pressed to find enough money for a cup of coffee, and we slept on the floor of the Gay Centre in extreme discomfort. It was cold and most of us were inadequately dressed. This was not good news since our ultimate destination would be Scandinavia – in winter. The first night was worse than uncomfortable. The Centre boasted a large, well-equipped kitchen. Closer inspection revealed, however, that it had not been used for some considerable time – it was also bereft of anything obviously resembling food. A pleasant young Swede called Lars, a strict vegetarian, had a particularly nasty experience. Hungry and desperate, he found a large jar of peanuts on a dresser in the kitchen. He had eaten quite a quantity of them before he noticed that the jar was alive with maggots; he vomited for hours.

Maureen Oliver

After spending another night sleeping on the floor, I found I was expected to speak on radio via the telephone at 7am... It was the worst talk I ever gave in my life - I could barely utter a coherent word. That evening we managed to get invited to a gay club, found the prices completely beyond us, kicked up a scene, and were summarily evicted. On our next, and last night in Zurich, I managed to collect enough money to buy the ingredients to cook a huge quiche to feed everyone on the bus. It was much appreciated; it seemed my maternal skills were not entirely defunct. However, we were fast becoming hobos, and hobos with attitude at that.

We left Switzerland and traveled through Germany, eventually arriving in Munich. The Gay Centre in Munich was small, but pleasant. In most of Europe – except Scandinavia – the lesbians and gay men did not mix at all. Lesbians were, for the most part, separatist and would have nothing to do with anything male whatsoever. So the Munich Gay Centre consisted of some rather nice, gentle gay men who treated us well. However, we found ourselves sleeping on the floor yet again. The performances and my rallying speech went down well, but we were vagabonds now, and were up for anything. There was a curious fashion at the time of wearing stolen symbols from Mercedes cars as jewellery. There were a lot of Mercedes cars in Munich. The lesbian band sported some trendy ornaments when they gave their performance that night, and so did I. Years later, I would suffer pangs of guilt about it, but back then it just seemed like innocent fun.

There was an incident. The members of the women's band and I, tired of male company, decided to find a lesbian club. We found one and almost gained admittance, until that is, Debbie, one of the band members was spotted. Debbie was black. The door of the club was firmly closed on us – we screamed and kicked the door and yelled abuse but to no avail.

The band, Mouth Almighty, four women singers with their roots firmly in Punk, wore their hair in great tangled spikes around their heads. They told me they achieved the effect with soap – Imperial Leather was the best. They decided to give me something of a makeover and soon my hair stood out in black tentacles around my pale face. I liked it, and I kept it that way for the duration of the tour. The members of Mouth Almighty were Scottish football fans, Celtic supporters and they were delighted I was a lapsed Catholic; it helped me fit in. The comedy trio, three gay men, consisted of an established couple in their early thirties and a younger guy called Ashley. They did a routine in which they would blow condoms up to a gigantic size put them over their heads then prick them with a pin so that they exploded. It was all good fun and in the cause of safer sex.

The members of the Munich Gay Centre had a problem. Dachau, the Nazi Concentration Camp, was nearby. They were distressed by the fact that there was no acknowledgement that homosexuals were among those who died there in WW2. We discussed what to do about this. We wanted to have some sort of demonstration, but it would have to be very low key. We didn't want to cause any kind of offence or disturb the atmosphere of grief and remembrance. We decided to hold a small candlelit ceremony next to the official memorial. They say that no birds sing there, and it was certainly true that day. An eerie silence permeated the camp. We had our memorial service, took some photos and walked around in the gathering gloom. Then a guard started to shout that we should get out as it was closing time. We didn't hurry. Somehow it didn't seem appropriate. Then he came up very close to us and yelled that if we didn't get out straight away he would lock us in. We were all in tears on the journey back to Munich.

After Munich we journeyed on to Nuremberg. In many ways it was a beautiful city, but our reception was far from lovely. The first thing we encountered was anti-Dutch feeling. The English and Scandinavian members of the tour were treated OK in the shops and bars, but the Dutch aroused loathing and people were openly rude and insulting to them. That night we were to do our stuff in a large hall. It was not a Gay Centre and was open to the general public. A Dutch woman was translating – this didn't go down well. It was an uncomfortable experience and worse was to follow. A group of skinheads started to jeer at us and make Nazi salutes. Our scandalized audience reacted angrily; scuffles broke out and the meeting ended in confusion.

We packed up and left, heading for West Berlin – the route would take us through communist East Germany.

We crossed the border in mist-shrouded darkness and were directed to a hut where we were to be issued with passes. Our passports were scrutinized and one guy, the oldest member of our party, had the misfortune to be wearing a luxuriant wig at the time. The guards got very excited, waving their arms about and saying that his passport photo looked nothing like him. Finally, one of them grabbed the wig and pulled it off the head of the hapless man. We were issued with our credentials and sent on our way. East Germany was in total darkness – a bleak and forbidding terrain, but we soon cheered up when we found that alcohol was incredibly cheap. The bus was duly stocked with every kind of strong drink known to humankind, and we were in ebullient mood as we drove through the night towards the Brandenburg Gate, Checkpoint Charlie, and entry into West Berlin.

By the time we arrived at the venue we were so intoxicated we could barely stand. Our Dutch tour guides were horrified and wanted to stop us going on stage. It's important to point out that we had a passionate commitment to our cause and that we had set out on this journey with high ideals and dreams of building international solidarity. We had not started out as vagabond alcoholics; that happened after a few weeks of living on the road. So, there we were in Berlin – a scruffy, unkempt mob pickled in booze. It was a poor state of affairs. Somehow through the haze of drunkenness we knew we had to sober up and do our stuff. We drank copious amounts of black coffee, studied our scripts and eventually lumbered into the spotlight. It didn't go too well... My speech was weak and one member of Mouth Almighty fell off the stage in a drunken stupor. We didn't exactly cover ourselves in glory. We got, undeserved beds for the night in Berlin but, chastened by our tumble from grace, didn't take advantage of the local night life but opted for the chance of a good night's sleep instead. People just did not understand us. The woman who put me up was annoyed by my using her washing machine and draping damp clothing all over the radiators in her flat, but I hadn't had the opportunity to clean up my act for a while and so the next morning, after the blissful luxury of sleeping in a real bed I showered without her permission too. The next day I was booked to speak in the Reichstag – quite an honour. I was a member of a panel of 'experts' quizzed by a large audience; the conference roundly condemned the British legislation as homophobic and pernicious.

Throughout all of this I was becoming more and more convinced of my own importance; my drive and purpose distorted into arrogance verging on the grandiose, and I became increasingly obsessed with mysticism and the occult. The Goddess featured in my thoughts a great deal; though I didn't speak about her I began to secretly commune with her. It was probably around this time that it occurred to me that I might be the Goddess's chosen one – sent to right wrongs and save the world… I regularly read the Tarot cards for my companions; it helped idle away the tedium of endless travel and reinforced my notoriety.

Hamburg – at first sight just a busy port with a thriving shopping centre, yet our venue that night would be in the heart of the porn industry – the Reeperbahn. Everything went well. There were a lot of women there that evening, so I tailored my speech to concentrate on the plight of lesbian mothers and the phrase 'pretended family relationships'. After the meeting I found myself surrounded by lesbians who had lost their children through the German courts. We hugged and wept – it was an emotional evening.

That night I went on a tour of the bars with the three gay comics. I don't remember too much about it, except that one of the men had a heated discussion with me about which one of us had the hairiest legs. We ended up taking down our trousers in the middle of the Reeperbahn - watched dispassionately by a group of assorted prostitutes – I don't remember who won the contest. That night I was due to stay with the other lesbians at the home of a local woman. I got there late and rather the worse for wear, and found everyone else curled up in sleeping bags on the living room floor. I complained loudly that there was no room for me, not even a pillow on which to lay my head. At that point, our hostess appeared and said quietly that I was to sleep with her – it was a capacious, and comfortable, bed and I lay awake briefly wondering if I was meant to make love to this woman or not. What was the etiquette for such a situation? I didn't wonder long however because I very quickly fell into a profound sleep. The woman seemed very put out the next morning...

We continued our journey, heading north to Denmark, our next venue would be in Aalborg, unsurprisingly it was growing very cold and snow

BEING ICARUS

was now fluttering past the grubby windows of the bus as we sped on. The driver of the bus was a venerable old hippie who had brought with him three dogs for some unaccountable reason... These dogs had a habit of wandering off and getting lost – hours could be spent looking for them. So we drove into Aalborg – hippies, activists, performers and animals – quite a travelling circus. We explored the city, found second-hand shops and kitted ourselves out with warm clothing and boots – just as well, it was very cold. The venue was a large, municipal building set back in its own grounds, it had a bar with people seated around tables – cabaret style. We were very well received and treated. The Danish lesbians and gays had given up their apartments for us and we were given keys and free access to their homes. I stayed with Dennis and two comedians in a comfortable flat full of stripped pine and polished floors. It was warm and stocked with food and coffee, bunk beds, everything except a bathroom. There was a toilet but no bath or shower. I kept searching for one hopefully but, as it transpired, the people of Aalborg used public bathhouses – there was one at the end of the street. We behaved well in Denmark perhaps because we were shown respect, the local people were charming and considerate and we left the city cleaner, calmer and better fed than we had been for some time. We journeyed on towards the ferry to Gothenburg – and Sweden.

The crossing was fairly unremarkable save that we once again had a source of cheap alcohol and settled in to some serious drinking. The dogs proved something of a nuisance during the voyage; our driver had distaste for putting animals on leashes, so they wandered about the boat causing mayhem. Once we reached Gothenburg, the inevitable happened. Sweden had strict anti-rabies laws and the dogs were impounded. Their distressed owner said he would have to accompany them back to Holland, so we were held up in Gothenburg for a while – we had to find someone else to drive the bus... The thing I remember most about Gothenburg was that I was now obsessed by the Tarot. Someone had sold me a new set of the cards and I constantly read them for other members of the crew and for myself. It was about this time that I began to feel a sense of impending doom. I became convinced we were heading for disaster. My companions scoffed at my fears – but I was quite sure, it was all in the cards...

From Gothenburg we travelled to Norway, to Oslo. The land of the midnight sun – though autumn was turning to winter as we approached the city; the sun hung huge and red, low over spectacular scenery of snow covered, pine clad mountains. The people of Oslo had laid on a meal in our honour in a smart restaurant. I had been booked

BEING ICARUS

to return home after Hamburg, there was supposed to be a car waiting to drive me to Belgium for the sea crossing. There was no car, and frankly, by this time I was not inclined to return home. The tour had become my world, and, with all its discomforts and difficulties, I had a feeling of belonging and of acceptance – this was a drug to someone who had suffered a lifelong sense of isolation – and I was hooked.

A woman called Mellita inspired some rivalry, she was expected to take over from me as official speaker of the tour; no doubt I saw her as a usurper. The rivalry usually took the form of friendly banter but at the meal we found ourselves both attracted to the same woman. The woman, a smart and wealthy Norwegian lesbian, chose me and, later, after a successful performance, I found myself sharing her bed. Her magnificent home was perched on top of a mountain and the lights of Oslo twinkled beneath us under a velvety, indigo starlit sky, as we lay entwined together. The lovemaking was warm, intense and wonderful and I was desperately in need of it after so long on the road.

The next morning we were up at dawn, just as that enormous sun was rising above the horizon; long shadows cut ultramarine streaks through the gilded snow. My lover gave me strong coffee and a little breakfast and suggested that we ride down the mountain together – on her pushbike. This was exhilarating and terrifying, the bike slid rapidly, and dangerously, over the icy paths and at one point – I was perched on the crossbar – we hit an obstacle and I flew backward over my friend's head landing several feet behind on the, all too solid, ice. We laughed uproariously. I was bruised and scratched but otherwise unharmed and so, joyfully, we rode together, still full of the heat of passion, into Oslo. I said a tearful farewell and the bus moved on – back to Sweden, and Stockholm.

BEING ICARUS

Chapter 4
Disaster.

The bus headed relentlessly on toward Stockholm. My anxiety reached fever pitch as I dealt the Tarot cards time and time again. "The 'Tower of Destruction' ", I moaned aloud, "'Death', all will end in chaos – in disaster!" By now the crew just sniggered or asked me to 'put a sock in it', but I was convinced, nothing could shake my belief that we were heading for trouble. And I was to be proved right.

We arrived at the RFSL – the Gay Centre in Stockholm, tired, the worse for wear and desperate for drink. The Centre was truly magnificent. In the whole of Europe we had seen nothing like it. The floors and huge elaborate staircases were of solid marble and they shimmered in pearly splendour; one could almost see Fred and Ginger waltz across the vast and splendid entrance hall. The place exuded and dripped wealth and status. We were taken to the homes of refined gay men who offered us comfortable beds for the night and fed us fine food. Then we returned to the Centre for the night's performance. Mellita spoke well as I remember, and, later we all sat in the bar together somewhat disconsolately. Alcohol was very expensive and we were broke. I remember that the five of us – the band and myself - bought one large beer and tried to drink it through straws. The theory was that the straw would cause the alcohol to hit the spot and the effect would be multiplied. It didn't seem to help much. The evening wore on and I was looking forward to a comfortable night's sleep, when all hell broke loose.

There was a tremendous commotion, screaming, yelling and the breaking of glass. Two of the members of the comedy trio were fighting with some Swedes on the staircase and one of the lesbians from the band – a small woman named 'Red' was being pursued by the barman. I learned later that a woman had grabbed a bottle of whiskey from behind the bar. The barman had beaten Red and her head had been pounded against the marble while she lay surrounded by whiskey and broken glass. Two of the comedians had come to her rescue and an almighty 'punch up' ensued. The police were called and came, complete with huge truncheons and jackboots, they pulled two of the women into a room and blocked access to it with more police. Terrible screams issued from the room and me, and other women, tried to get in to help. I did manage to gain entry at one point and saw a police officer astride one of the smallest of the women pulling her arms up behind her back. She was screaming in agony. I ran over and exerted all my force trying to lever his hands away from her wrists before being forcibly ejected from the building. At this point I 'lost it' and started yelling hysterically. At that precise moment, the entire plate glass window of the RFSL shattered into a million pieces. I was handcuffed and thrown into a police car and soon found myself frightened, confused, arrested and charged.

I was charged with breaking the window although I had been 6 feet from it at the time. While in the police station I was threatened and intimidated. At one point an officer ordered me to get down on the ground – I had been perched on a wooden bench – or he would beat me to a pulp. I cowered terrified in a corner, utterly confused. Later, the lover of the woman believed to have stolen the whiskey, joined me. We were not allowed to talk to one another but it was comforting not to be alone. I was charged, and after several hours my passport was taken and I was warned not to leave the city. I was then released into the darkness of a Stockholm street. It was about 4am. Some of the members of the crew were waiting nearby and took me to an all night café where I found the other members of the tour. Two of the women from the band had been held in custody and the hearing was to be the next morning.

We turned up at court, and gasped in horror as the women were brought to the dock battered, bloody and bruised. They had been badly beaten. The magistrate ruled that they should be detained pending trial. The trial was to be in a fortnight. We were homeless, penniless, in a strange city and two of us were in jail. I was charged with criminal damage and not allowed to leave the city, as was my companion at the police station – Stella. It was now November, bitterly cold and dark most of the time. The local houses had Advent candles shining from their windows – Christmas was approaching – but it seemed there was no inn or stable in Stockholm for us. We huddled in corners in cafes anxiously debating what to do. At this point the local Women's Centre stepped in. They were angry that the men of the RFSL had called in the police – believed to be notoriously brutal – rather than dealing with the situation themselves. Local lesbians and feminists came forward and we were eventually given the loan of a spacious apartment. Meanwhile, the mainly male, remaining members of the bus tour held a vote as to whether they should continue the tour or stay with us. They voted to travel on without us. We felt betrayed.

The following weeks would be a strange and desperate time for the small group of women left behind. The charges against Stella and me were eventually dropped for lack of evidence but we stayed in Sweden in support of the imprisoned lesbians. In any event, we had no means of returning home. It occurs to me now that we could have approached the British Embassy for help but we never thought of doing that. We remained

BEING ICARUS

dependent on the local women's network for help and support. Here in Stockholm, in the gathering gloom of winter, I would soon encounter Swedish political activists – and genuine witches.

I took refuge in alcohol and the weaving of spells. The Goddess now spoke to me in my despair and called me to do her bidding.

A woman called Katherine – a Norwegian nurse – called often at the apartment carrying food, bottles of whiskey and cans of beer. One afternoon I read the Tarot for her, she leaned over me while I did so, her body touching mine, and I sensed her desire. Katherine became a very important guest. Her visits with food and drink were vital and we all felt indebted to her. One night I had drunk the best part of a bottle of whiskey and started vomiting in my sleep. I was dragged to the bathroom by the other women, stripped and held, still vomiting, over the bath; I had been in danger of choking to death. I was a mess. My mind was in disarray and I now believed I was the chosen one of the Goddess, she told me so frequently, yet at the same time I felt terrible guilt and despair as wasn't it after all, all my fault? And there were other voices, voices taunting me, voices deriding me, voices condemning me. In all of this I struggled to survive, struggled to keep hold of some kind of reality. Katherine was a Pagan – a Goddess worshipper – a witch, and she introduced me to other witches in Stockholm. Many of the Stockholm witches – male and female – were involved in some sort of political activism. I've never been quite sure why the connection. At one political meeting, ostensibly called to discuss police brutality, I found myself surrounded by witches.

We visited the women in prison and soon knew the date of their trial. On the night before, a local coven were to cast spells for a favourable outcome. I was invited to participate and I turned up at a small apartment in the centre of town nervously anticipating being expected to cavort about naked. It was a decorous affair however. One of the witches was sick and lay in bed throughout which rather spoiled everything, as the exact number of participants was vital. We performed some rituals, lit candles and chanted spells. I remember being irresistibly amused by the fact that the warlock and leader of the group, a large middle-aged bearded man, wore a green leaf incongruously pinned to his tangled grey hair.

The morning of the trial dawned. I was called as a witness – so did not get to hear the testimony of the others – but I was informed that the barman 'Christian' had confirmed the theft of the whiskey and that a policeman had had his finger broken by one of us. I realized that I could have been the culprit. I had tried to force away the hand of the man who had been hurting my friend. She had been screaming in agony and it could have been me, or one of the other women – who knows? He had been so brutal; I couldn't feel much sympathy for that broken finger as I gave my evidence. In spite of the efforts of that local coven, and all my prayers and supplications to the Goddess – the women were found guilty and sentenced to a month's imprisonment. We sobbed as they were led from the dock. They would serve a further two weeks. What would we do at the end of that time? We had no way of getting home, no money, no resources at all. We seemed doomed to trudge the dark icy streets of Stockholm forever like some accursed shades of our former selves.

.

We kept ourselves busy. I became involved for a while with groups of local activists campaigning against the police. I was given a poster picturing a Turkish immigrant who, it seemed, had been beaten beyond recognition following an arrest. It was a very disturbing image. I sent it back to the campaigners in Britain, hoping to rally support. But that support would never come. As far as the lesbian and gay community back home was concerned we were an embarrassment, a disgrace, and nobody wanted to know. I suppose that wasn't totally surprising given that the events in Stockholm were triggered by someone stealing a bottle of whiskey from a gay bar - no one seemed to care, however, about the disproportionate violence and brutality that had been meted out. No one in Britain anyway – we had supporters in Stockholm after all.

After another two weeks, the imprisoned women were released. It was an emotional reunion; we hugged and kissed them warmly and then went back to the apartment for some serious partying. However, our benefactor now needed it back and we had nowhere to go and no money. Unknown to us however, the remaining members of the Bus Tour had been rallying support for our cause in Denmark and Holland. A Dutch lesbian collective had managed to raise enough money to pay for our flight back to Amsterdam. From there we would travel back home. We were delighted; at last we were on our way. We spent an evening at the home of Katherine in the suburbs of Stockholm. It was a Swedish festival and all the food had to be yellow or orange. There were a lot of lentils but it tasted good. During the evening it became transparently obvious that Katherine had taken quite a fancy to me. Back at the apartment it was agreed that I should 'reward' her by spending the night with her before our departure, and I did. The sex was pretty good and I found Katherine a surprisingly imaginative lover, though she toyed with restraint and pain as a vehicle for pleasure. This didn't faze me however; in fact I quite liked it. I was driven to the airport the next morning, just in time to catch up with the other women and board

BEING ICARUS

a plane for Amsterdam.

I had been worrying about my daughters this whole time. They were eighteen and seventeen, but still in school. They had no money – how had they been surviving? I should have been home within three weeks but it would be nearly three months before my eventual return. The voices I heard roundly condemned me as totally evil except for the messages from the Goddess who whispered to me of the great things I would achieve.

The Amsterdam lesbians greeted us with open arms and in festive mood we headed for an artist's collective in a converted warehouse on the bank of one of the canals. Here we would spend the night – fuelled by copious supplies of hashish provided as gifts. It was a strange night. We all sat cross-legged in a circle passing spliffs around and drinking hot, sweet, black coffee. The drug had a powerful effect on me. I started to see the other women as scheming bitches trying to bring about my downfall. I fell into a morose silence watching them, convinced a plot was being hatched. I had acquired, in Norway I think, a black beret with an enamel red star brooch pinned to it, and I found the red star missing. This all seemed to be part of the plot, and I brooded distrustfully in a corner eyeing the other women with something approaching real malice. Of course the voices chipped in with endless warnings. "Be careful Maureen, they want to destroy you" and "They will kill your spirit and you will fail in your mission". By now I knew that my 'mission' was to do the Goddess' bidding, I knew myself to be her High Priestess – the chosen one – elevated above all of humankind and destined to save the world. The next day we flew back to London.

BEING ICARUS

Chapter 5.
A Chill Wind Blowing...

In the women's toilet at Heathrow I studied my reflection in the mirror with alarm. My black, spiky hair was now splashed with a shock of white and my face was lined and drawn. I seemed to have aged 10 years in the last few months. Anxiously, I headed for my home in the South London suburbs.

My children were upset and angry. Falteringly I tried to explain about the arrests and the impossibility of my getting home sooner – but it was useless. All of my paintings had been stripped from the walls, a broken window had been recently mended and the place seemed cold and desolate. It turned out that my daughters had had one hell of a party while I was away. Flocks of teenagers had attended and things got quite out of control. A window was broken and the floor had been littered with bottles, cigarette butts and the odd condom. My father had answered their pleas for help and had provided them with some cash and my ex had paid for the broken window to be mended. Rent and bills had, of course, not been paid; bailiffs pounding on the front door had only been repelled by the prospect of being savaged by the family dog. The two girls shouted at me crying. Weak and nervous after my experiences, I could not deal with the situation and fled to the house of

49

a gay activist friend in North London. I hid out there for a week or two trying to regain my strength. Eventually there was a tearful reunion with my family and some kind of normal life resumed – briefly.

I decided to travel the country telling the true story of the European Bus Tour against Clause 28 and visited a few venues. I think people were more shocked by my weakened state and appearance than anything but there was still not much support for the arrested and imprisoned lesbians; we were all seen as a disgrace to the campaign. The consensus was that it was best that the whole thing should be forgotten. Perhaps it would have been best, after all, but I felt myself to be on a mission to tell the story of the brutality of the Swedish police and the cold-blooded attitude of the Stockholm Gay Centre – the RFSL.

The events in Stockholm cast a long shadow and I was in poor spirits – weak, confused, depressed and periodically hallucinating. There was to be yet another blow. OLGA was being sued by another gay organization. It transpired that our young, inexperienced treasurer, who had been keeping the office running while Dennis and I were away on the Bus Tour, had published a letter disputing the right of two actors, one of them greatly celebrated, to call themselves gay activists. The actors were major players in the campaign and had initiated a lobbying group and rival organization – pouring considerable money and resources into it. Apparently, they were enraged by the letter and went straight to a solicitor. They claimed libel. We were informed that we would be sued for 'every penny we had' and could lose our homes and everything we possessed. This worried us – until we realized that none of us possessed very much at all. We were all three penniless, lived in rented property and had no regular income. We had nothing for anyone to take. We were still very concerned since it seemed that the costs could be levied from the organization's membership. Eventually, we met the aggrieved activists around a negotiating table and the case was dropped in return for an official apology. I breathed a sigh of relief and attempted to pick up where I had left off and start some serious campaigning.

I struggled to keep working and did a reasonable job of running the OLGA office, though my energy levels were now low and everything seemed a great effort. Then the letters started arriving…

Katherine had not, at the time, left a lasting impression. She was rapidly becoming a fading memory. The first love letter was therefore something of a surprise, but as time went on and letters kept arriving I started to depend on them; they became a balm for my battered self-esteem and sustained me through a dark depressing time. Her letters were both warm and passionate. She spoke of how heartbroken she was that I was no longer in Stockholm but in London, out of reach of her embraces. Her desire seemed to burn from the pages and I began to bask in the belief that she longed for me to return. There was a popular song at the time: 'Forever Autumn', its haunting refrain went − '...because you're not here', Katherine claimed to be playing this music endlessly, thinking of how she missed me so much. I fell for it and dreamed of being back safely in her arms.

Christmas came and went and, one day, a letter arrived containing a plane ticket for Stockholm dated for mid-January. I had no money − a not unusual state of affairs − but, at the designated date and time, I boarded a flight for Sweden. All I had in the way of cash was a solitary ten-pound note and I was flying to one of the most expensive countries in the world. Katherine had woven her spell and I was rushing to my fate, heading back to the city I had grown to loathe believing that she loved me. I was mesmerized by a vision of being cherished and wanted and was plunging headlong into a bizarre and cunning trap.

In my confusion I took the wrong train to the airport − the slow one instead of the express - and arrived just as the Stockholm plane was taking off.

BEING ICARUS

I yelled and cried at the airline desk that it was all the fault of the railway system. They relented and gave me a seat on the next flight but Katherine would have been waiting to meet me. I managed to phone and leave a garbled message for her with an irritated Swedish airport clerk who admonished me for my lack of language skills. A few hours later my plane touched down in Sweden and I rushed through customs looking desperately for Katherine. We soon found each other, she was clearly annoyed by my late arrival but greeted me warmly, saying mysteriously that there was someone she very much wanted me to meet. She took me back to the former scene of the crime, the RFSL, the Stockholm Gay Centre, where I encountered 'Penelle' for the first time.

Penelle was clad from head to foot in black leather, from her boots to the cap on her head; she also wore studded wristbands and a great set of keys jangling from her belt. She was a sturdy muscular woman with cropped blonde hair and sharp, blue eyes and, as I approached, she looked me up and down in a predatory fashion that I found unnerving. It seemed Katherine had made another conquest. I had a ticket to return to England in ten days time and ten pounds in cash. I felt helpless and devastated but if I thought for a moment that Katherine was no longer interested in me I was very wrong.

The two women took me back to Katherine's apartment where a precise set of arrangements awaited my arrival. I felt completely powerless. Like a lamb to the slaughter I allowed them to do whatever they wished. A bath was run and sprinkled with very particular herbs and Katherine undressed me and bathed me. Then I was led into the bedroom and put to bed. It was essential, said Katherine, that I spend this night alone, and, as I fell into a deep, possibly drugged, sleep they left taking Katherine's huge black dog with them. I slept for a very long time, probably 24 hours, before they returned. The talk was of the Craft and I was, literally, spellbound as they performed complex rituals. It was much later that I fully realized the significance of those rituals - the symbolic binding with rope and the Fivefold Kiss. They had initiated me as a witch.

The days and nights that followed were strange indeed and, ultimately I was stranger than they had bargained for. Penelle was a sadist as well as an erstwhile practitioner of the Occult and intended to seduce and control me. I was easy meat. Soon I was on the receiving end of mingled pleasure and pain at her hands and became a sexual pawn in an elaborate game played out between the two of them. The sadism was more than play and at one point they thought I had died. I lost consciousness and Katherine couldn't find my pulse for 20 minutes. Where now was the

BEING ICARUS

feisty self-opinionated campaigner? In the midst of all of this my psyche was a battlefield. I heard constant voices and the Goddess appeared to me in visions and trances. I saw myself circling around her gigantic frame constructed of ice, I experienced myself as Lilith, the true first woman, giving birth to the whole human race in agony and in another vision I saw myself as a Priestess of the Hearth in Ancient Greece and knew that that was my first incarnation. Strange things began to happen. At one point the room tilted; it seemed as though reality itself would slide away. The Goddess spoke through me saying she sought 'vengeance' and that she/I was on the 'Pathway'. I became a channel for her. I experienced falling through the earth's crust into a deep underground chamber and being attracted to a door with radiant light streaming from it – I wanted to open the door believing that my dead mother waited on the other side, but I was warned not to and brought back. Anxiously, Katherine stuffed dirt into my mouth and made me eat it, saying it would 'ground me'. Other witches were brought in to observe, but they all left, frightened.

Finally, Katherine and Penelle huddled together on their bed begging me not to come near them. They had intended to subdue me and use me for sex but they had unleashed something quite awe inspiringly deep and dark and they were terrified. I believe they were incredibly relieved when they

eventually put me back on the plane for Gatwick.
But what had happened to me?

BEING ICARUS

Chapter 6.
Famous and Frantic.

With a painful flap of his waxen wings, Icarus headed for the burning Sun and self-annihilation.

I returned to London a changed woman. My previous low mood had been replaced by a nervous manic energy, I saw myself as all-powerful, after all didn't I know that I was the Goddess' chosen one, her High Priestess of the Sacred Flame? I kept the knowledge to myself; this stage in my mission was not the right one in which to reveal the truth. I often heard the voice of the Goddess instructing and supporting me, though sometimes her tone could change and she could be mocking, cruel and angry. Other voices derided me but I reasoned that these were demonic in origin and that I mustn't heed them. Only the Goddess must be obeyed and only she was worthy of my love and devotion.

I had a lover in Scotland - Helen, a young woman with a Dutch artist mother. Helen lived in Edinburgh and was an artist herself. We had a love of art in common, and I should have done everything in my power to hold on to a relationship that was both passionate and warm. However I took the overnight bus to Scotland in a weak and confused state of mind. I told Helen something of what had happened in Stockholm – of the sadomasochism and witchcraft. She looked at the marks on my body, close to tears. She talked to me all through the next night about women victims of sadists. She said their apparent compliance hid depression and instability. She knew two such women who spent their time in and out of psychiatric units. Her wise words fell on deaf ears; I was communing with the Goddess and lost to reason. The next day I travelled back to London. Gradually, and quite horribly, our relationship would fall apart. Eventually Helen would be unable to take any more and would abandon me to my fate. Who could blame her? Later, losing control, I would slap her in a sudden fury in the unlikely setting of the Royal Academy of Arts Tearooms... I would beg forgiveness, but by that stage it was all over between us. Later still matters would take a bizarre turn that would become a key point in my descent into total confusion and madness.

Meanwhile I continued to campaign with ferocious purpose. I was flying high, very high, though now it did not feel good at all. I was possessed by a manic, driven energy and a sense of inner desperation and I threw myself into my work with intense abandon.

Early in 1989, the International Lesbian and Gay Association, ILGA, were meeting in Amsterdam. I determined to attend and to let people know about the cruel treatment meted out to the Bus Tour

BEING ICARUS

lesbians. It would be tricky as only invited speakers were allowed on the platform and ILGA owed much of its funding to the wealthy Swedish group – the RFSL. I went with Helen as her parents lived in Amsterdam and it was home to her. We stayed in an apartment left empty while the lesbian owners were on holiday elsewhere. I started out in a quiet way, attending the conference in an informal capacity. While there I was delighted to meet up again with the four women from the lesbian band – Mouth Almighty. We spent some time together in the bar plotting. It was decided that the only way to get to tell our story was for me to single handedly 'storm the platform'.

The following day, at a given signal, I rushed forward, evading security, and leapt onto the stage. I grabbed the mike and began to speak, my voice shaking with emotion. As the stewards went to grab me and drag me away, the delegates called for me to be allowed to finish what I had to say. Floris was there, quietly orchestrating things from the back of the hall – he gestured to me to slow down, I had been rushing my words nervously. I steadied my pace and gradually got into my stride. As I detailed the events of that night in Stockholm some of the lesbians in the meeting were clearly moved. When I finished there was a call for a vote of censure against the Stockholm police and the RFSL. The result was close, the conference was almost split 50/50, but the RFSL won the day, though I believed mine to be the moral victory.

Attitudes to me were hardening, and I was gaining a reputation as 'mad, bad and dangerous to know'. To my horror I was told that the formidable Lisa, present at the conference, had made a complaint. Apparently, she believed I was harassing her with continual 'silent' phone calls. The dye was cast, the label stuck.

On New Year's Eve, in the apartment in Amsterdam, Helen and I had a fearful row. The women owners of the apartment were coming back unexpectedly and we had to get out. I suggested that we stay with Helen's parents but the idea didn't go down too well.

We were 'rescued' by my friends from the Bus Tour, the Dutch hippies. They invited us to stay in the huge, ancient house in central Amsterdam that they squatted. We arrived with our bags and were allocated a large room lined with aged mirrors, dusty and smelling of decay. We accepted the offer eagerly, and settled down to stay the night.

I slept only fitfully. Very early in the morning Helen left and I stayed alone in the great bed as a grey dawn tried unsuccessfully to penetrate the gloom. Slowly I became aware of presences gathering in the half-light. Faces materialized from the haze; floating above me they pressed on me and peered at me. Pinioned on the bed I lay petrified. At last I was able to get to my feet. I tore out of the room, rushing down to the communal kitchen in panic. One of the hippies told me calmly that he wasn't at all surprised; the house had been owned by a seventeenth century physician and that particular room had been his mortuary.

Back in London, my first arrest took place outside the South African Embassy in early 1989. In order to fulfill my belief in solidarity, I had linked OLGA to those behind the 24-hour picket of the Embassy – the Revolutionary Communist Group. Here I encountered hard line activists prepared to take risks and well schooled in political rhetoric. I began to attend the picket regularly and often spoke from a soapbox, my voice ringing out across nearby Trafalgar Square, startling tourists and pigeons alike.

A major action was planned. Douglas Hurd, the then Foreign Secretary, was to visit the Embassy, and meet with white South African dignitaries - perpetrators of apartheid. We were determined to give him quite a reception.

A large crowd of protestors had gathered in the wintry twilight. It was about 5.30pm and the police were out in force keeping the demonstrators safely penned behind barricades. Slogans were yelled fervently, but I itched to do more. Six of us, all but myself sturdy young men, plotted to leap the barricades and run towards Mr. Hurd. We never discussed quite what we intended to do when we reached him. Just as he got to the door of the Embassy, at a given signal, all six of us vaulted over the barricades and started to run at speed. The police, taken unaware for a moment, soon rugby tackled all five of the men and brought them to the ground. I ran on, almost invisible in my black dungarees. I got to within three feet of the Foreign Secretary, screaming at the top of my voice and energetically waving a placard, before I was grabbed and tossed over the barricades like a rag doll. I was thrown into the back of a police van with the others and we were driven the short distance to the cells at Bow Street. The sergeant who charged me said I was guilty of attempted murder. I was taken into a room and strip-searched by a woman PC. As I removed my clothing I asked the PC if she enjoyed her work. "Yes", she replied breezily, "I do, I *really* do". That over, and my being found to have no concealed weapons, I was chucked into a cell and left alone. I wasn't, to my great relief, charged with attempted murder but a mere public order offence. I was booked to appear before the magistrate the next morning. Once there, I eloquently disputed the claim of the arresting officer that I had screamed obscenities on the basis that no feminist would ever use such language. The Goddess quietly expressed her approval as I did so. The magistrate looked a little puzzled but, although I was found guilty, I was let off with a reprimand. I was free to fight again.

A major opportunity for fighting the good fight soon materialized. A new group – ACT UP London – based on a successful AIDS campaigning group in the States, was set up and I soon found myself elected 'Action Convener'. My job was to orchestrate imaginative protests. We took direct action to a new level – we made an art of it. A large percentage of the members of ACT UP were artists of one kind or another. Our numbers included designers, artists and writers plus Jimmi – a rock star then at the height of his fame. The mixture was seasoned with a scattering of left wing political activists, notably the fabulous three. These last were a team of dedicated communists who lived together in a run-down flat off East Street market. Their task seemed to be to recruit ACT UP members to the party, and influence policy and decisions. They were skilled, trained infiltrators.

It was around this time that I was contacted again by my old friend Floris from Amsterdam. He wanted to organize a protest against the Viennese authorities. A group of protesting lesbians and gays had been badly beaten by the police. Floris told me he had a great idea. I arrived with a small group of campaigners and listened to his plan and it was certainly a crazy one. The idea was to go to Amsterdam Central Station and handcuff ourselves to an inter-Europe express train as it was about to leave for Vienna.

So it was that I found myself handcuffed to the front of that massive engine with only seconds to spare before it roared into life. This was some experience. By now I was very aware of the importance, and desirability, of press coverage and a motley crew of photographers were assembled on the station platform; as the cameras flashed I believed my end had come but just in time the Dutch police arrived. They looked rather puzzled. "Why did you do this?" they asked me. I explained the situation in Vienna. "Oh", they said amiably, "that's really terrible" and they handed back the cuffs and chains smiling indulgently. I was bruised and covered in oil from the engine but excited and triumphant. Another battle, another victory. The Goddess was delighted with me; I was fulfilling my destiny.

ACT UP's first direct action in London was to block the road at the busy Elephant and Castle roundabout during the morning rush hour. We believed the Department of Health to be there, unfortunately it had moved by then, but, nevertheless, the demonstration had quite an impact. We caused utter mayhem and came close to being attacked by angry motorists. I chained myself across the entrance to the building. Floris had given me the handcuffs used on the Amsterdam Station demo and I put them to good use. I developed a tendency to chain myself to any and every object in sight – a tendency that would later afford me some notoriety. We blocked the road with a huge banner. The press coverage was very good. Our protest was a response to the fact that people living with AIDS were being denied the financial help they needed. The rules for Sickness Benefit were that a low rate was paid for the first 6 months, consequently people sometimes died before they could get the money they desperately needed. This regulation was later reviewed and the needs of seriously ill individuals were eventually taken into account.

So ACT UP London was successfully launched. It became a sexy campaign. Our much sought after black T-shirts displayed shocking pink inverted triangles and the slogan 'Action = Life'. Soon they were to be seen everywhere in the bars and clubs. We even made the front pages of tabloid newspapers. I was interviewed on television and radio, and ACT UP members travelled the country raising awareness.

I didn't confine myself to ACT UP and joined Anti-Racist Anti-Fascist Action spending time confronting the likes of the British National Party. I also continued to speak on the picket of the South African Embassy and on one occasion I stayed up all night painting a huge sheet of black fabric with the portraits of Nelson Mandela, Steve Biko and other legendary heroes of the fight against Apartheid. The next day I took it to the Embassy and a large group of us sat down in Trafalgar Square with the painting stretched out across the busy road. We were dragged away by the police, but I would have none of that and repeatedly threw myself back into the traffic. Then, without warning, I jumped into the path of an oncoming car – it couldn't have stopped – but two police officers, one a WPC, dragged me away just in time. The young WPC, sweating and exhausted, looked at me in horror – "You're old enough to be my Mother," she gasped, and I was.

For ARAFA, I helped organize a demonstration outside a National Front pub in Kings Cross. We stood yelling slogans as leather-jacketed fascists glared back at us. They were lined up threateningly outside the pub – the police struggled to separate the two factions. Six of us went inside with a petition demanding that the National Front be barred. Enraged bigots yelled abuse and spat at us. When I appeared there were screams of 'Hope you die of AIDS, gay bitch'. If the police hadn't been there I think we would have all been torn apart.

BEING ICARUS

At another demo for ACT UP, outside the Department of Health – this time the correct building in Whitehall - we held a large banner across the pavement to protest against the unfairness of the benefits system. At first it was a decorous affair, but then, a few of us, Jimmi included, lay down in the road covered by the banner. The press, out in force, enthusiastically snapped away at the rock star activist. The police were flinging people onto the pavement with some abandon. Filled with revolutionary zeal I grabbed the banner and raced out into the road, the banner flying behind me like a mighty flag. Wildly high, enthusiastic and impervious to danger, I tried to throw myself into the path of an oncoming bus. Once again, I was plucked from certain death by two officers and was unceremoniously thrown into the back of a waiting police van. Bruised and with ripped clothing I screamed slogans to the sound of wild cheering from the assembled crowd of protestors - until the doors slammed upon me and I was driven to Bow Street yet again. I was charged with obstruction and walked free from the court once more – fired with a burning desire to repeat the experience. I was becoming truly manic, and what was that death wish all about? Yet many saw me as a hero…

It was in April that Helen finally dumped me. I simmered with rage. Fortunately she was in

Edinburgh and I was home in the London suburbs. I sat up into the early hours making a tape of the most angry, bitter and aggressive songs I could find. I intended to post it to Helen as a way of communicating my anger and grief. It was a strange night; I poured my venom into the music. The tape was an act of revenge. I didn't post it; in the cold light of morning I threw it aside. However, soon afterward I would have occasion to remember that strange night and those violent feelings. A few days later, I had a call from a terrified Helen. Strange things had been happening in the house in Edinburgh; rumbling noises, flashes of light, the rooms shifting, shaking and tilting. Eventually, Helen, her landlord and the other residents had fled into the night. They sought sanctuary with a friend, a professed white witch. Her voice shaking, Helen asked me to stop 'hexing' her house. I was frightened and amazed. How, I asked, could it be that I could cause these things to happen when I was hundreds of miles away? However, when it transpired that the night of the strange phenomena in Edinburgh was the very same night that I had poured my bitterness and anger into making the 'hate tape' I was shaken to the core. Had I really caused those things to happen? A month later, around the time of my birthday, I had another call; Helen's new lover, a woman called 'Che', had started to speak in 'my voice', yelling and screaming demonic abuses. Yet again strange psychic phenomena had taken place in the house in Edinburgh. This time I was told a warlock and two covens of witches, one in Scotland and one in Cornwall, had been contacted to 'seal my power'. Helen invited me to speak to the warlock, but I declined. I was now absolutely terrified. What on earth would my fate be with two covens and a warlock sending negative energy my way?

My experiences became darker and more intense. I frequently heard condemning voices and began to have nightmarish visions. Only the Goddess stood by me. Only she told me how much she loved me and how precious I was in her sight. How I had a special mission to fulfill for her. How I would save the world. People were not to be trusted. I had to be very careful. I read the Tarot Cards endlessly, trying to discover who my enemies were. Nothing was as it seemed to be. I began to read the signs, to see secret motives behind apparently harmless words and actions. I was being persecuted; there was danger all around. "Be careful", said the voices, "They are out to destroy you".

Meanwhile, ACT UP staged one of its most effective and imaginative demos. At that time, the authorities refused to acknowledge that men in prison were having sex or that that some prisoners were injecting drugs. Because condoms and clean needles were not provided, AIDS was spreading through the prison population at an alarming rate. We designed and built a gigantic working catapult and took it to Pentonville. Once there, we set it up in the street outside and catapulted condoms, clean needles and information leaflets over the high wall of the prison. Cheers of appreciation went up from the prisoners in the yard on the other side of the wall. We got plenty of press attention, the action was filmed for TV and I was interviewed. The police were out in large numbers; black police vans lined the street, but miraculously no one was arrested that day.

It was around that time that Susannah, the female member of the communist trio, began to court me. I found her attentions flattering; I had become isolated and solitary. Soon I found myself drawn into that select group. Increasingly fragmented by inner turmoil, I was unable to discriminate between genuine love and friendship and political opportunism. I was Susannah's lover for a while. However, she didn't know what she was taking on. All too soon I would be overwhelmed by mental distress and would sink into confusion; hallucinating and frightened I would try to cling to her for support. It must have been difficult and after a while she left me. In any case, I was of no use to her by then – political or otherwise.

I became increasingly 'out of control' and could no longer hide my mood swings and my, often weird,

BEING ICARUS

behaviour. On a small demonstration outside the Virgin Music Store I was expected to play the role of an aggrieved mother. I was to complain to the manager about the offensive lyrics of a popular song. However, when I started to act the part, rage took over. Instead of merely complaining to the unfortunate manager, I screamed violent abuse at him. Unable to stop, I was dragged away by another protestor before I could do any substantial damage. I had totally 'lost it'.

Chapter 7
The Descent.

Icarus, his melting wings tipped with flame, began falling, falling from light into darkness. From the heat of the Sun he fell, till at last he drowned in the cold depths of the waiting sea.

In the late summer, I travelled to Amsterdam once more with Ian, our treasurer. We were to run a stall at an event in the city and would stay with Floris. It so happened that some other women I knew were staying nearby, and they invited me to a lesbian club. At the club, I found myself dancing with my old rival, Mellita from the Bus Tour. We had plenty to drink and I felt elated and convinced that Mellita wanted to spend the night with me. She came back to Floris's house with me, and we cuddled for a while on my makeshift bed in the basement. I felt powerful, virtually omnipotent. I told her I didn't *work* for the campaign and in fact I *was* the campaign. She leapt up and said she'd find somewhere else to sleep. A sudden uncontrollable rage possessed me. Yelling and screaming, I grabbed her and threw her down on the bed. She fought back and I slammed her against the wall in a fury. She was trembling with fear. Then, my senses returned and she ran crying for help locking herself in the bathroom. Floris was up and trying to calm the situation. By this time I was sobbing for forgiveness. I was in torment.

BEING ICARUS

What had I done? The voices chimed in, echoing my thoughts, "What have you done now, Maureen? What *have* you done?" Dawn came up and Mellita left. I wept, and tore my hair - I no longer knew myself. Was I a monster? I was kicking and throwing myself about in my anguish and Floris was afraid for his priceless antiques in their glass-fronted cabinets. Eventually he calmed me down a little. He said that Mellita might be able to forgive me someday, but would I ever be able to forgive myself? My unpredictable moods and actions had reached crisis. Nothing would ever be the same again.

When I got home, my mind was in turmoil. As the days and weeks went by, I tried to track my moods - rage, despair, sadness, elation and godlike omnipotence. I seemed to ricochet from one to another without warning. Worse still, they seemed more than mere moods; I experienced them as separate 'entities', as totally different beings. The voices I heard told me I was possessed by an Angry Goddess called 'Anu' and a sad frightened child called 'Marina'. They warned me of some terrible fate - of impending doom. Still, my Good Goddess spoke to me of the wonderful mission I was on, how I would save humankind and how I was her chosen representative on Earth. But sometimes my Good Goddess would turn her face and the Angry Goddess would take over. Her voice would then assume a threatening tone. I was ringed by intrigue and danger. My former friends were plotting against me. Yes, I was sure of it, the voices warned me to be careful. There were forces out there that wanted to destroy me utterly.

One day I phoned my younger brother who lived in Bath. He was something of a mystic, a successful Tarot reader and Astrologer. I told him about the evil mocking voices and he was very concerned. As a result, he sent me a secret Talisman with strict instructions to show it to no one but to meditate on it in private. He assured me this would help. For a while I derived comfort from it, but then my mood changed again. I felt compelled to carve the magical letters in the Talisman on my arm with a sharp blade. I thought I would be better protected from evil. I must have misunderstood.

I travelled with a group of colleagues to a meeting in an old farmhouse. The house was set amid beautiful scenery in the heart of the Sussex Downs. It had been thought that the weekend trip would be a way of combining business with pleasure. I have no recollection of what that business actually was, or indeed who those colleagues were. I just remember that the house was very old, in a state of disrepair, and isolated. We talked into the night. I was left alone in what served for a living room, to sleep on the couch in front of the dying embers of a coal fire. There was

BEING ICARUS

a worn old mirror, framed with curved shapes that culminated in two peaks. They looked like devil's horns. I looked at the mirror in the dim glow of the dying fire, and saw a huge eye staring back at me; a vast, solitary green eye. I shuddered and turned away. I tried to sleep and then something was pressing down on my body, touching me, all over me, I couldn't move and I couldn't make a sound. It was on me, it was in me, it took me and I could barely breathe. When it was gone I lay quietly sobbing. I knew I had been visited by a devil, a demon from Hell. Then the mocking voices started again. The next morning I wandered around the farmhouse for ages wearing nothing but a sheet wrapped inadequately around me. I was lost in a waking nightmare. My companions were shaken by my strange behaviour. Someone took me home.

It was the autumn of 1989 and I was rapidly descending into madness. My gift for public speaking had left me; either I would babble inanely, mistakenly believing I was making clever and incisive comments, or I would stumble haltingly and find it difficult to find any words at all. Sometimes people laughed at me. I experienced rejection again and again, and because I did not understand that I was doing anything wrong I felt alienated and afraid. I believed I was surrounded by conspiracies. Even those I had accounted friends seemed to be plotting against me. In order to defend myself against the evil forces threatening me I adopted a hostile attitude. There was almost no one I could trust.

Jenny and Lisa invited me to an event at their home in East London. It would be a gathering of luminaries. The great and the good from the lesbian and gay rights struggle would all be there. I was deeply fearful and confided my fears in my, by now, long suffering sidekick, Dennis. I begged him to go with me because it was bound to be a plot after all. Imagine my confusion when, at the close of the evening, I found myself praised and feted for my part in the 'struggle'. Jenny and Lisa led the applause and I was kissed and hugged by celebrities and activists alike. Briefly I wondered if all my fears were unfounded. However, by the time I reached the local station to start my journey home, I knew the plot must be deeper than I had at first thought. "Take care," said the voices, "they are out to kill you."

Autumn turned to winter; there was to be an international conference in Brighton organized by none other than Mellita. I was invited to speak and also present would be my old friend Floris and the Norwegian woman with whom I had had that glorious but brief affair in Oslo. I arrived with a small, loyal group of supporters and flew into a rage at the outset because a feminist magazine had failed to print an article of mine. The voices

BEING ICARUS

told me it was all part of the plot against me and I believed them. I had been badly beaten on a recent protest and my leg was swollen, bruised, and swathed in bandages making walking painful and difficult. When I arrived at the hall where the meeting was to be held I was very loud and positively rude to the assembled delegates. I decided that I needed some vodka. I hadn't indulged in serious drinking since the Bus Tour, but, at that moment, it seemed to me that only alcohol could hit the spot. Under some pretext I collected money in a hat, then went out and bought the vodka. I drank most of it myself. Later, I believed my performance and speech were exemplary, but in reality I was probably incoherent. Floris was deeply upset, he tried to take me aside and make me see reason but I couldn't see that I was doing anything wrong.

That night there was a benefit party at a local club. I went along, convinced that I was irresistible to all women. I wandered around the tables in a predatory fashion but was rebuffed in no uncertain manner. I started to feel afraid; what was happening to me? Later, in another club, I was mocked and cruelly laughed at by a large group of lesbians. I began to weep hysterically and my little cohort of gay men took me back to the flat where we were to stay the night. They made me coffee and tried to talk to me. I was lost. Nothing made any sense at all. Why were people rejecting me? I felt totally confused and the voices chimed in warning that they were all out to destroy me. Frightened, humiliated, and feeling totally alone I took the train home in the morning.

I kept trying to work. The few people who still cared, told me to take a holiday, to get some rest. But I didn't know how to stop. My daughters were very worried as I had lost a lot of weight and, on the rare occasions I was at home, they tried to get me to eat. At a student conference in Blackpool I aroused derision yet again. There had to be a reason, clearly people were plotting to destroy me. I read the Tarot cards over and over again trying to identify my enemies but soon I suspected everyone. The Goddess communed with me frequently. Now she began to tell me that there was something of a change of plan. She wanted me with her in Paradise and in order to do that I had to become 'pure spirit'. I didn't comprehend it fully but I was becoming suicidal.

By December, in a sense, my fears were proved right. The other members of ACT UP wanted me to go. After all, I was now something of a liability. A week before Christmas there was to be a meeting. I read the cards yet again and saw the 10 of Swords. "Swords are in your back", said the voices, "they want to kill you." As I walked down to the Lesbian and Gay Centre, I repeated Hail

BEING ICARUS

Mary's endlessly. I needed protection.

When I walked into the meeting room it was as though I had walked into a nightmare. Familiar faces had become horribly distorted monstrous masks. Someone started to say how the group wanted to separate from OLGA. I knew then I was totally rejected. I ran out screaming and a gay friend took me home with him. When I woke up the next morning I saw my dead mother looking at me with a worried expression on her face. The Angry Goddess took over and the voices insisted that I was totally useless and a waste of space. I went into the kitchen and found a large knife and was trying to slash my arm with it when my friend came into the room. He got the knife away from me but afterwards fled the house. Fortunately he called a lesbian friend of mine who came and rescued me. She got me to stay at her house for a few days. Then, when I was rested, and a little calmer, she took me home to my daughters. It was almost Christmas. I remember asking why there were stalls selling decorations and a man dressed as Santa - it made no sense to me.

My daughters took care of me over the festive period but early in January there was a benefit party for OLGA and ACT UP. I wandered around seeing conspiracies everywhere. Some friends took me home with them for the night. I was being very abusive so they were walking ahead of me angrily. One of them, an American woman called 'Stacey', turned round and confronted me. I saw her as an enormous serpent rearing up at me. Enraged I thought that I'd like to slash the serpent open and visualized myself doing so, but then she was Stacey again and I began to weep uncontrollably.

Peter, a gay friend who had moved to Brussels, invited me to stay with him for a few days. I had phoned him and, worried, he paid for my flight. I managed to get lost in the city when I first arrived, but got a taxi to his house and soon fell into his comforting arms. He cooked me a lot of meals and talked to me for hours. He also bought me paints and paper and encouraged me to do some creative work. I painted a huge, bird of prey swooping down and grabbing me up in its claws; it was a recurrent vision. I would talk to tormenting voices through the long nights, sometimes yelling at them; my friend couldn't have got much rest. All too soon though I was back on the plane heading for London. Once there I again tried to connect with my campaigning and ended up getting lost in my own city while trying to make my way to yet another protest meeting. I ran frantically through the streets convinced that the devil was chasing me.

Clearly I could go on no longer. One day, feeling calmer than usual, I decided to see my GP,

BEING ICARUS

thinking maybe a few pills would help. In the event, I saw a locum. The woman looked at me dispassionately as I sobbed out my story. I told her I was afraid I was being pursued by the devil. "Yes," she said, "you probably are. Gay people are often mixed up in the Occult". This confirmation of my fears was not what I needed and I froze in horror. She was telling me about a minister she knew who could exorcize me, leafing through my medical notes as she did so. She obviously came upon my previous psychiatric records because her tone suddenly changed. "I am going to refer you to a psychiatrist," she said abruptly, "You should hear from him in a couple of weeks".

So it was that I found myself subject to a psychiatric assessment and interviewed on a cold day in late January 1990. As I tried to tell my story coherently, the consultant and his registrar – a redoubtable woman – discussed suitable drugs over my head. "Haloperidol do you think?" "Perhaps Largactil – or Stelezene – or both." I was told to attend the local psychiatric day hospital and turned up one clear frosty morning. It seemed a strange place to me. People just sat around blank faced, making fluffy soft toys, cutting out pictures from magazines or smoking obsessively in a designated corner. I was given Largactil and Stelezene and soon I started to feel woozy and thick headed. However I kept myself together by writing everything down in a small, black

81

notebook. Much later I learned that this was a mistake; it was deemed to be evidence of paranoia. I stayed in touch with my Good Goddess – she was very concerned about my fate. "Be careful," she warned, "they will turn you into ashes here". On my third visit to the day hospital, I found myself unceremoniously bundled into a taxi with a nurse escort. I was driven 10 miles out of town to Warlingham Park Psychiatric Hospital; a forbidding place. It was originally a Victorian insane asylum.

BEING ICARUS

Chapter 8.
Drowning.

It seemed to me I had arrived at the very portal of Hell. The nurse who admitted me, a capacious and kindly woman, asked me questions about my life, marital status, children and employment history in a slightly bored, toneless voice. Then she asked, "Religion?" I launched into an impassioned monologue, fervently describing the true nature of the Great Goddess – the Mother of All. I explained that God was really female and preaching the contrary view was, in fact, a patriarchal lie, about how the Goddess had contacted me, her High Priestess, with messages about my mission on earth and my eventual home with her in the afterworld. I detailed the revelations I had had from her and spoke of wonders and secret knowledge. I explained how the Goddess herself had told me I was her High Priestess – a sacred role. I was so close to the Goddess I was semi-divine myself. I informed the nurse about how the Great Being now expressed a desire for me to become 'a creature of pure spirit'. She wished me to abandon the semblance of an earthly form altogether so that I could be with her forever in Paradise. After some time, I paused to draw breath. "Right," said the nurse in a monotone, "I'll put you down as a Non-Conformist then."

Maureen Oliver

I was left to the tender mercies of a new psychiatrist. She seemed kindly and started by giving me a very thorough physical examination. I thought her rather attractive. She then ran through a breathtaking list of questions, making notes as she did so. After this, she told me firmly she believed I was suffering from Schizophrenia. As my mind struggled to cope with this, she comforted me with the news that there were medications that would help and I would feel 'better' soon.

I was introduced to a young, male nurse, whom I assessed, correctly, to be gay, and was told that he was to be my 'Primary Nurse' and that if I needed anything I was to talk to him. He was a pleasant personable fellow and asked me if I'd like some toast since I had missed 'Tea-time'. I nodded feeling rather numb and confused and sat down at a Formica-topped table in the eating area. When the toast came I ate a little and then wandered off for a while. When I returned I found a large, grubby looking man finishing off the last of my toast. "Hungry," he informed me abruptly and shuffled away fairly quickly.

I soon adapted to the hospital regime and rapidly learned which patients it was OK to approach, and which ones it was definitely best to avoid. At first I used to hover near the door, clutching my coat and my old derby hat, waiting for a chance to escape. However, it wasn't long before I observed the fate of those who had tried to do so - they were returned to the ward by the police like so much lost property. Sometimes they were handcuffed and then they were dragged away to the 'locked' ward where I was told they would be incarcerated for a very long time. So I abandoned my escape plans and tried to 'fit in'. I soon discovered, to my initial dismay, that the lavatories had no locks and that the bathroom door had to be kept wide open. Apparently a woman had managed to commit suicide by slashing her wrists in the bath. Nurses would visit us while we bathed and sometimes converse amicably. We were under observation but I got used to it. My younger daughter brought in paints, brushes and paper and I spent hours painting pictures of the Goddess, the All-Seeing Eye, angels falling from grace and sometimes demonic, grimacing faces. The Goddess was beginning to despair of me. Her voice became tediously repetitive as she constantly warned me "they will reduce you to ashes in this place. They will destroy you", but I now felt powerless, after all what could do about it, and what on earth could I achieve here anyway?

I did make a couple of friends in the hospital. One of them was a man in his late thirties; a recovering heroin addict, and the other was a girl of seventeen who had slashed her arms almost to ribbons. The young girl used to play loud rock music all day and I would dance frantically around the 'dayroom' waving my arms frenziedly, crawling under tables and jumping onto furniture. Sometimes I would practice Yoga and demonstrate headstands and various convoluted positions with considerable pride. This amused some of the patients and infuriated others. The nurses were a little concerned. It was hard to know what to do with my energy in the confined space of the ward so for the first few weeks I would pace rapidly up and down for hours. The sleeping arrangements consisted of long dormitories; one for the men and one for the women, but I didn't do a lot of sleeping. I'd get up and go downstairs, looking for cigarette butts to smoke, listening to the voices.

After 3 weeks I was allowed to go outside accompanied by my nurse – that pleasant gay man. We had some interesting conversations whilst traversing the grassy terrain surrounding the hospital. After another week or so I was allowed to go to the patient's café by myself. This was a tremendous treat. There was cheap coffee and cigarettes that you could buy individually if you had very little money and sweets and pies and a pool table too. I took to wearing brightly coloured plastic bangles given me by another female patient, someone else gave me some frilly pajamas and we all had a great variety of pills of many sorts and in various colours. We lined up for them dutifully several times a day – the nurse would watch us closely to see that we swallowed them and didn't hide them under our tongues in order to spit them out later. My lovely gay nurse spent much time explaining to me that I had a disease - an illness called Schizophrenia – and that I was not being chased by the devil or spellbound by witches. He told me that if I took the pills I would soon feel very much better but that I'd have to take them for the rest of my life "like a diabetic has to take insulin". I was soon convinced of the efficacy of the pills but less enthusiastic about forfeiting my belief in the power of witches, demons and that old Goddess.

I spent two months in Warlingham Park Hospital before being discharged to day care and home. My eighteen year-old daughter's boyfriend had moved in with her in my absence and just as well - she needed all the support she could get. I was quite a responsibility for one so young and her older sister was away at university. She was now doing a full-time course at an art college however, and, after I was discharged from day care, time seemed to drag; I missed my former active life as a campaigner and moped around the house occasionally listening to voices. The friends I had had when I was an activist, only months ago, had all but melted away. They had visited me in hospital a few times at first, but when I didn't soon return to my old self, they stopped coming and I didn't hear from them any more. One day in late spring, I decided to look through the phone book for something, anything I could find, somewhere I could go and meet people. I knew of the Mental Health Charity – Mind - and found they had a day centre in Croydon. I had to get myself referred by a social worker but that was not difficult, and I soon found myself among a large crowd of other people with mental health problems – people like me. I made friends there, discovering a small, close-knit group of lesbians who spent a lot of time in the Pool Room. One of them interested me very much and soon Brenda and I became lovers.

Unfortunately for me, owing partly to being prescribed too many 'side effect' pills, and partly due to depression after a hopeless attempt to reconnect with my former life, I found myself back in the day hospital treated with increasingly large 'depot' injections of a very powerful drug – Modecate. 'Depots' were humiliatingly administered via a needle into the buttocks and I had to drop my pants on a weekly basis. The effect of the drug was devastating and I became withdrawn and totally lacking in motivation. It was as though the life force had gone out of me. My lover stayed with me through seven years of this. Without her, and the love of my daughters, I think I would have killed myself. I was deep in despair but the pain was locked up inside; the drug made it impossible for me to express my feelings, and to

BEING ICARUS

others I just appeared blank - empty.

Epilogue.

Seven years later, I found the strength to refuse the Modecate. It was as though a light went on somewhere. It was grudgingly agreed that I could go back on Stelezene tablets for a trial period. Slowly, very slowly, I started to become myself again. I began to communicate a little and even made some crude attempts at painting and drawing. Gradually I came back from the dark. I became more assertive; sadly my relationship – based as it was on my partner being in a caring role – began to founder and finally broke down when I was on my sixth, and, to date, last hospital admission. However, Brenda and I are still closely linked in a warm and loving way that transcends friendship.

Newer medications became available. They still had side effects – massive weight gain for example – but they freed me further; I started to paint and write seriously. In the late nineties I became a campaigner yet again as chair of a local group of psychiatric survivors fighting for rights and better conditions.

In September 2000, I was on holiday with my elderly father on the island of Malta. I was stressed and tense as I had recently had my meds changed and it hadn't gone too well. At that time, I still, rather half-heartedly, subscribed to a pagan

BEING ICARUS

belief in the Goddess and various ill-assorted 'New Age' ideas. On the second night of my stay, I was sitting in my hotel room feeling rather bored. Then, I heard a soft gentle voice speak in my mind. The voice identified himself as Jesus Christ. I didn't want to listen, but he spoke of love and how he had been waiting for me all this time. "Go to the Bible," he said, and, sure enough, there was an English Bible in the room. "Go to the Bible and read." I opened the Bible at random. It fell open at the parable of the Good Shepherd. Then I knew what he was saying to me. How I had been that lost sheep all of these tumultuous years and how he had sought me out. I started to weep and determined that somehow I would find my way back to the Church. I didn't have any idea how, and I didn't believe that someone like me could really be *allowed* in the Church, but I determined to try.

At the moment I am seeing a psychologist who tells me I suffer from dissonance. I think I could give lectures on the subject. Here I am, trying to be a practicing 'good' Catholic while also believing in Lesbian, Gay, Bisexual and Transgender Rights. I still see myself as a feminist and, after all, I *am* a mad woman to boot.

Back in April 2001, I put on a solo exhibition of my new paintings at the Diorama Arts Centre in Central London. Everyone I knew came to the preview; my family, old friends, friends from the psychiatric 'system', my friend Peter from Belgium and, of course, my ex-lover and best friend, Brenda. I was nearly 54, my struggle was not yet over, but I had hope and a head full of dreams and life beckoned.

Maureen Oliver, 2007.

www.ingramcontent.com/pod-product-compliance
Lightning Source LLC
Chambersburg PA
CBHW031220290326
41931CB00035B/599